I0706568

PNEUMONIA PREVENTION COOKBOOK FOR NEWLY DIAGNOSED

Delicious Recipes, Lifestyle Tips, Meal Plans, Expert Guidance, And Proactive Strategies To Boost Immunity And Strengthen Your Respiratory System

DR. ERIC TRISTAN

CONTENTS

Copyright © 2024, By Dr. Eric Tristan

All Rights Reserved

All rights reserved. No part of this book may be reproduced, distributed, or transmitted in any form or by any means, including photocopying, recording, or other electronic or mechanical methods, without the prior written permission of the author, except in the case of brief quotations embodied in critical reviews and certain other noncommercial uses permitted by copyright law.

DISCLAIMER

The information provided in this book, is intended for informational purposes only. The content is not intended to be a substitute for professional medical advice, diagnosis, or treatment. Always seek the advice of your physician or other qualified health provider with any questions you may have regarding a medical condition. Never disregard professional medical advice or delay in seeking it because of something you have read in this book.

The author of this book has made reasonable efforts to ensure that the information provided is accurate and up-to-date at the time of publication. However, the author makes no representations or warranties of any kind, express or implied, about the completeness, accuracy, reliability, suitability, or availability of the information contained within these pages.

Any reliance you place on the information provided in this book is strictly at your own risk. The author shall not be liable for any loss, injury, or damage arising from the use of this book or the information contained herein.

The mention or reference to any individuals, products, websites, organizations, or other names within this book does not imply endorsement by the author. The inclusion of such references is solely for informational purposes and does not constitute an endorsement or recommendation.

Furthermore, the author disclaims any association or affiliation with any individuals, products, websites, organizations, or other names mentioned in this book.

It is important to consult with a qualified healthcare professional before making any dietary or lifestyle changes, especially if you have a medical condition. Each individual's health situation is unique, and what works for one person may not work for another.

Again, the information provided in this book is not intended to diagnose, treat, cure, or prevent any disease or health condition. Always seek the advice of a physician or other qualified health provider regarding any medical questions or concerns you may have.

Thank you for your understanding and for taking the necessary precautions when considering the information presented in this book.

ABOUT THIS BOOK

This "Pneumonia Prevention Cookbook" is an essential reference that offers a thorough examination of how to enhance respiratory health by implementing lifestyle modifications and dietary modifications. This book commences with a perceptive Introduction that establishes the foundation for a thorough examination of the complexities associated with pneumonia prevention. It proceeds to explore the central theme by providing a comprehensive explanation of the foundational principles of Understanding Pneumonia, thereby enabling readers to comprehend the significance of tailored nutritional interventions.

The following chapters provide an overview of Nutritional Foundations for Respiratory Health, promoting the consumption of a diet that enhances the body's resistance to respiratory obstacles. This book "Constructing a Pneumonia-Resistant Diet" and "Incorporating Immune-Boosting Foods" provide pragmatic advice on how to prepare meals that target pneumonia prevention specifically. The investigation into Key Vitamins and Minerals for Respiratory Wellness enriches the reader's comprehension of vital nutrients that are indispensable for the preservation of pulmonary well-being.

A holistic approach is promoted by Hydration Strategies for Lung Health and Balancing Macronutrients for Immune Support, which highlight the interdependence of nutrition and respiratory health. By incorporating Herbs and Spices for Respiratory Wellness, the reader gains an additional resource that supports the development of a lifestyle resistant to pneumonia.

In addition to theoretical guidance, this cookbook offers practical instructions in the form of Cooking Techniques for Nutrient Retention, which effectively applies the information gained to the preparation of routine meals. Meal planning for pneumonia prevention guarantees the adoption of a respiratory-friendly diet sustainably and practically.

This book's final sections, titled Recipes for Respiratory Health, Snack Ideas for a Strong Immune System, and Beverages for Respiratory Support, provide an extensive assortment of palatable and healthful alternatives. In addition to dietary considerations, this book emphasizes the significance of upholding a healthy lifestyle, which includes factors such as exercise and respiratory wellness, sleep hygiene to support a robust immune system, and stress management to prevent pneumonia. As a cohesive unit, these chapters establish a comprehensive structure that enables readers to take an active role in protecting their respiratory health by employing practical strategies and well-informed decisions.

CHAPTER ONE

Introduction

As a respiratory infection that impacts the airways, pneumonia is an important issue in global health. Although medical interventions and vaccinations are essential for pneumonia prevention, dietary decisions can also strengthen the body's immune system against the disease. The primary objective of The Pneumonia Prevention Cookbook is to offer pragmatic and palatable strategies for improving respiratory well-being. By acquiring knowledge about the fundamental principles of pneumonia and adopting a diet that is abundant in essential nutrients, individuals can proactively promote their overall health.

Comprehension Of Pneumonia

Pneumonia is distinguished by the presence of pus in the air sacs of one or both lungs; its etiology typically involves infections caused by bacteria, viruses, or fungi. In vulnerable populations, severe cases of the disease, which is characterized by symptoms such as fever, congestion, and difficulty breathing, can be fatal. Preventive measures encompass the maintenance of a strong immune system and the reduction of pathogen exposure.

Aware of the multifaceted nature of pneumonia prevention, this cookbook acknowledges this. It underscores the importance of adopting a comprehensive approach that integrates dietary strategies with medical advice. Instead of substituting established medical practices, the cookbook functions as an auxiliary resource that leverages the potential of nutrition to improve respiratory health as a whole.

Fundamentals Of Nutrition Regarding Respiratory Health

A nutritionally dense diet serves as the fundamental building block for respiratory well-being. Essential nutrients, including zinc, selenium, and vitamins A, C, and E, are critical for safeguarding the respiratory tract and bolstering the immune system. An assortment of lean proteins, fruits, vegetables, and whole cereals guarantees a dietary regimen rich in nutrients.

This cookbook offers recommendations for choosing foods that are abundant in anti-inflammatory and antioxidant compounds. Berries, verdant greens, nuts, and seeds are included. Omega-3 fatty acids, which are abundant in flaxseeds and fatty seafood such as salmon, have anti-inflammatory properties that are advantageous for respiratory health. Aware of the nutritional underpinnings necessary for optimal respiratory function empowers individuals to make well-informed decisions regarding their daily dietary selections.

Developing A Diet Resistant To Pneumonia

Practical recipes designed to strengthen the body against pneumonia are included in the cookbook. Dishes are formulated utilizing components renowned for their anti-inflammatory and immune-boosting attributes. As an illustration, a meal comprised of a vibrant salad comprising kale, spinach, and berries would be abundant in vitamins and antioxidants. Soups that incorporate garlic, ginger, and turmeric highlight components that are renowned for their potential antimicrobial and anti-inflammatory properties.

Promoting digestive health is the incorporation of probiotic-rich foods into one's diet, such as fermented vegetables and yogurt. Enhancing the functionality of the immune system, a healthy gastrointestinal microbiome provides an additional barrier against respiratory infections. The cookbook supports the notion that a diverse and vibrant assortment of foods is essential for obtaining a wide range of essential nutrients.

The Integration Of Immune-Boosting Foods:

Specific foods are widely recognized for their ability to enhance the immune system, and the cookbook deliberately integrates these foods into palatable recipes. Citrus fruits, renowned for their substantial vitamin C content, are utilized extensively in fruit salads and invigorating beverages. Lean sources of protein, such as poultry and legumes, supply the immune system with vital amino acids.

Additionally, the cookbook presents infusions and herbal beverages containing immune-boosting botanicals such as elderberry and echinacea. These beverages not only provide a soothing sense of warmth but also administer a potent quantity of compounds that promote health. By integrating these food items into their daily dietary regimens, individuals can proactively bolster their immune system, thereby establishing a robust defense mechanism against respiratory infections such as pneumonia.

In summary, this Pneumonia Prevention Cookbook functions as an all-encompassing manual for incorporating nutritional principles into a more comprehensive approach to respiratory health. While recognizing the significance of traditional medical treatments, it emphasizes the value of a nutritious and balanced diet. Through a comprehensive comprehension of pneumonia, adoption of nutritional foundations, construction of a pneumonia-resistant diet, and integration of immune-boosting foods, individuals can actively promote their health. This gastronomic methodology not only imparts a gustatory aspect to well-being but also enables individuals to assume responsibility for their respiratory health via the decisions they execute in the culinary space.

An All-Around Strategy For Respiratory Health

As a respiratory infection that impacts the airways, pneumonia is a potentially fatal and severe condition. Although medical intervention is of utmost importance in the management of pneumonia, implementing a preventive strategy via a specialized cookbook can make a substantial contribution to respiratory health. This article delves into fundamental principles outlined in a Pneumonia Prevention Cookbook, with particular emphasis on the integration of essential vitamins and minerals, methods for maintaining proper hydration, achieving macronutrient balance, and consuming foods abundant in antioxidants.

Essential Minerals And Vitamins For Respiratory Health

It is critical to prioritize the consumption of specific vitamins and minerals to sustain a healthy respiratory system. Vitamin C, which is widely recognized for its immune-enhancing attributes, is indispensable in the prevention of respiratory infections, such as pneumonia. Strawberries, bell peppers, and citrus fruits are all excellent sources of vitamin C, which can be used to enhance the flavor and nutritional value of dishes.

Vitamin D is an additional vital nutrient that regulates immune responses to promote respiratory health. Sunlight, fatty salmon, and fortified dairy products are all excellent sources of vitamin D. By incorporating these components into a cookbook dedicated to pneumonia prevention, the nutritional composition of meals can be improved, thereby strengthening the body against respiratory hazards.

Trace elements such as zinc are essential for respiratory health and immune function. Incorporate zinc-rich foods such as lean meats, legumes, and seeds into recipes to guarantee a sufficient zinc intake. Seafood, whole grains, and legumes are all rich in selenium, which is essential for immune system health.

With an emphasis on these essential vitamins and minerals, the Pneumonia Prevention Cookbook endeavors to furnish nourishing, balanced meals that promote respiratory health as a whole.

CHAPTER TWO

Methods Of Hydration To Promote Lung Health

Although frequently disregarded, adequate hydration is vital for maintaining pulmonary health. Sufficient hydration aids in maintaining the moisture of the mucous membranes within the respiratory tract, thereby promoting the elimination of pathogens and irritants. It is crucial to incorporate hydrating foods and beverages into the pneumonia prevention cookbook.

Vegetables and fruits that are abundant in water, including watermelon, cucumber, and celery, not only aid in hydration but also supply vital vitamins and minerals. Soups and broths derived from transparent, fortifying liquids offer the added benefit of rehydration to those who are also in search of a comforting, warm meal.

In addition to increasing the diversity of a recipe, herbal teas, including peppermint and chamomile, provide additional respiratory benefits. By promoting overall lung health and soothing the respiratory tract, the warmth of these infusions can be beneficial.

By integrating hydration techniques into the recipe book, individuals can establish a comprehensive approach to respiratory health that underscores the critical role of fluids in bolstering the body's defense mechanisms.

Macronutrient Equilibrium For Immune Support

It is critical to maintain a balanced diet comprising appropriate proportions of macronutrients to bolster the immune system and mitigate the risk of contracting pneumonia. Fats, proteins, and carbohydrates each contribute in a distinct way to the maintenance of overall health.

Lean proteins, which are available in poultry, fish, lentils, and legumes, are rich in essential amino acids that support proper immune function. Incorporating a diverse selection of whole cereals into the cookbook guarantees a sufficient consumption of carbohydrates, thereby providing the body with a sustained supply of energy. In addition to supporting immune responses, healthy lipids, which are present in avocados, almonds, and olive oil, contribute to the overall nutritional balance of the body.

The primary objective of the pneumonia prevention cookbook is to achieve a balanced composition of these macronutrients, guaranteeing that users consume a wide range of essential nutrients that promote respiratory health and immune support. The compendium advocates for the consumption of whole, nutrient-dense foods to foster sustained energy levels and enhance overall health.

Incorporating Foods Rich In Antioxidants

Antioxidants prevent respiratory infections such as pneumonia by neutralizing free radicals and decreasing inflammation, both of which are critical functions of antioxidants. The cookbook on pneumonia prevention emphasizes the integration of foods abundant in antioxidants as a means to fortify the body's resistance against detrimental pathogens.

Berries, spinach, and tomatoes, among other vibrantly colored fruits and vegetables, are abundant in antioxidants such as vitamins A, C, and E. Nuts and seeds, sunflower seeds in particular, and almonds in particular, offer an additional antioxidant boost.

In addition to imparting flavor to dishes, the incorporation of herbs and spices, such as garlic, turmeric, and ginger, introduces potent antioxidants that possess anti-inflammatory attributes.

The promotion of respiratory wellness is facilitated through the utilization of antioxidant-rich ingredients in the recipes of the pneumonia prevention cookbook, which contribute to a palatable and health-conscious culinary experience. In addition to bolstering the immune system, these foods enhance the complex and multifaceted nature of the dining experience.

A Pneumonia Prevention Cookbook represents, in summary, a proactive and comprehensive strategy for promoting respiratory health. Through the consumption of antioxidant-rich foods, macronutrient balance, and the incorporation of vital vitamins and minerals, individuals can bolster their immune systems and mitigate the likelihood of contracting respiratory infections.

This cookbook not only emphasizes the promotion of health but also presents a wide variety of delectable dishes that enhance overall wellness.

Spices And Herbs For Respiratory Health

Not only have herbs and seasonings been utilized to impart flavor to food, but they may also provide additional health benefits. In the realm of respiratory health, specific spices, and botanicals are notable for their immune-boosting and anti-inflammatory attributes.

1. Turmeric, renowned for its bioactive constituent curcumin, exhibits formidable antioxidant and anti-inflammatory characteristics. It has the potential to mitigate inflammation within the respiratory tract, thereby potentially reducing the incidence of respiratory infections.

2. Oregano, which is abundant in compounds such as thymol and carvacrol, possesses antimicrobial and anti-inflammatory attributes. Oregano may potentially improve respiratory health and strengthen the immune system when incorporated into dishes.

3. Garlic contains the sulfur compound allicin, which possesses antimicrobial properties. Consistent ingestion of garlic has the potential to bolster immune function and aid in the defense against respiratory infections.

4. Ginger: Ginger's antioxidant and anti-inflammatory properties may be beneficial to

respiratory health. It has the potential to alleviate symptoms of respiratory infections and relieve irritation in the respiratory tract.

The inclusion of these seasonings and herbs in culinary preparations not only improves the sensory experience but also provides an additional barrier against respiratory ailments.

Techniques For Cooking To Preserve Nutrients

How we chop and simmer our food has a substantial impact on the preservation of essential nutrients that promote holistic well-being, including respiratory health. To maximize the efficacy of the Pneumonia Prevention Cookbook, it is critical to employ culinary methods that maintain the nutritional integrity of the ingredients.

1. Steaming: A method of preparation that is delicate on vegetables and proteins, steaming helps retain the maximum amount of nutrients. It is especially effective at preserving minerals and vitamins that are

water-soluble and contribute to a healthy immune system.

2. The utilization of minimal oil in sautéing is advantageous as it aids in the preservation of heat-sensitive nutrients. It is a flavorful and expedient heating method that improves the nutritional value of food without sacrificing flavor.

3. Slow cookery is a method that permits ingredients to percolate and harmonize flavors, all the while maintaining their nutritional integrity. This technique is highly effective in producing nourishing stews and soups that promote respiratory health.

4. Raw Preparations: The direct consumption of vitamins and antioxidants is achieved by incorporating raw fruits and vegetables into salads or munchies. Raw preparations are crucial for preserving the nutritional value of specific nutrients that are susceptible to depletion when cooked.

CHAPTER THREE

Meal Preparation To Prevent Pneumonia

The implementation of strategic meal planning constitutes a fundamental aspect of the Pneumonia Prevention Cookbook. A nutrient-dense and nutritionally balanced diet promotes overall health and may aid in the prevention of respiratory infections.

1. Incorporate Assortment of Vivid-colored Vegetables: Vegetables of various hues provide an array of antioxidants, vitamins, and minerals. The inclusion of an assortment of hues guarantees a broad spectrum of nutrients that bolster the immune system.

2. Lean proteins, including those found in poultry, fish, lentils, and legumes, offer vital amino acids that are indispensable for tissue maintenance and repair, including that of the respiratory system.

3. Whole cereals, including quinoa, brown rice, and oatmeal, are rich in essential nutrients, fiber, and complex carbohydrates. These factors support long-lasting energy levels and general well-being.

4. Probiotic-dense Foods: Fermented foods such as yogurt, kefir, and sauerkraut supply the gastrointestinal tract with advantageous bacteria, thereby promoting immune system health. Respiratory health is profoundly dependent on a healthy intestinal microbiome.

Dishes To Promote Respiratory Health

The creation of recipes that are tailored to promote respiratory health constitutes a fundamental component of the Pneumonia Prevention Cookbook. Two remedies that are intended to fortify the respiratory system are as follows:

1. Ginger-Turmeric Carrot Soup:

• Components:

• Carrots, vegetable broth, turmeric, ginger, garlic, and onion.

Instructions (•):

• In a saucepan, sauté the shallots, garlic, and ginger.

Carrots, turmeric, and vegetable broth should be added.

• Bring vegetables to a simmer until tender.

Blend until a uniform consistency is achieved.

Season as desired.

2. Salmon Roasted in Oregano with Lemon Garlic Quinoa:

• Components:

Quinoa, salmon fillets, oregano, garlic, and lemon.

Instructions (•):

Salmon should be rubbed with garlic, oregano, and lemon.

Salmon should be roasted until cooked.

Quinoa should be cooked with garlic and citrus.

Salmon served atop quinoa.

Snack Suggestions To Boost The Immune System

Snacking is an essential component in sustaining energy levels and supplying supplementary nutrients. Consider the following refreshment suggestions for respiratory health and a robust immune system:

1. YOGURT Parfait In Greece:

Greek yogurt layered with granola, berries, and a sprinkling of honey constitutes a delectable and immune-enhancing refreshment.

2. Nuts Spiced With Herbs:

Incorporate cayenne pepper, turmeric, and a pinch of sea salt into roasted mixed almonds to create a delectable and health-promoting refreshment.

3. Apple Slices Spread With Almond Butter:

• For a gratifying and nutritious refreshment, combine the protein and healthy lipids found in almond butter with the crisp flavor of apple slices.

In summary, the Pneumonia Prevention Cookbook adopts a comprehensive perspective on respiratory health.

Through the strategic integration of herbs and seasonings, the utilization of culinary methods that preserve nutrients, and the formulation of recipes and snacks that promote respiratory health, individuals can actively fortify their immune systems and mitigate the likelihood of contracting pneumonia.

By embarking on this gastronomic expedition, one not only provides nourishment for the body but also commemorates the delight derived from savoring flavorful, health-conscious fare.

Beverages Used To Support Respiration

The impact of the beverages we consume on our respiratory health can be substantial. Specific constituents can aid in the prevention of pneumonia and the maintenance of healthy lungs. Green tea, for instance, possesses anti-inflammatory properties and is abundant in antioxidants, both of which may promote respiratory health. By incorporating turmeric and ginger into smoothies or infusions, one can obtain immune-boosting and anti-inflammatory properties. Moreover, soups prepared in tepid broth, particularly those containing garlic and shallots, have the potential to alleviate respiratory distress while also supplying essential nutrients.

A decongestant effect can be produced by herbal infusions of peppermint and eucalyptus, which aids in the promotion of clear airways. Sufficient hydration is of utmost importance, and the consumption of diluted fruit juices, water, and herbal infusions can aid in the maintenance of ideal mucous viscosity, thereby promoting simpler respiration.

Upholding A Health-Conscious Lifestyle

Maintaining a healthy immune system is crucial for the prevention of pneumonia, and one's lifestyle decisions significantly impact this. Promoting overall health is possible through the consumption of a nutrient-dense diet comprised of an assortment of fruits, vegetables, whole cereals, and lean proteins, which supply vital vitamins and minerals.

Foods abundant in antioxidants, including verdant greens, citrus fruits, and berries, can aid in the fight against oxidative stress and strengthen the immune system.

It is crucial to restrict the consumption of refined foods, excessive sugars, and unhealthy lipids. The implementation of these dietary modifications aids in the regulation of body weight, thereby mitigating the likelihood of complications associated with obesity that may undermine respiratory well-being.

As smoking is a well-established risk factor for pneumonia, it is critical to avoid secondhand smoke exposure or cease smoking to prevent the disease.

Although water retention is frequently neglected, it is critical for the health of mucous membranes. Water aids in the regulation of respiratory secretions' viscosity, thereby averting their accumulation and impediment to clearance.

CHAPTER FOUR

Physical Activity And Respiratory Health

Consistent engagement in physical exercise is fundamental to optimal well-being, and it substantially influences respiratory health. Physical activity improves lung capacity, strengthens the respiratory muscles, and enhances cardiovascular health as a whole. Aerobic exercises, including but not limited to brisk strolling, jogging, and swimming, enhance oxygen exchange and blood circulation by stimulating deeper respiration.

Engaging in deep breathing exercises, such as tai chi or yoga, has the potential to optimize lung function and enhance respiratory efficacy. Additionally, these workouts facilitate relaxation, which can be advantageous in the management of stress, a well-documented contributor to immune system compromise.

Despite this, personalized exercise regimens must be adapted to the health conditions and fitness levels of each individual.

Seeking guidance from a healthcare professional or a fitness expert can be beneficial in developing an individualized exercise regimen that effectively considers the requirements of the person while maximizing the benefits of physical activity.

Sleep Hygiene For Immune System Strength

Optimal sleep quality is an essential element of maintaining a healthy lifestyle and is closely associated with immune function. The body performs vital physiological processes, including the secretion of substances that enhance the immune system.

Insufficiencies in sleep duration or quality may compromise the integrity of the immune system, rendering individuals more vulnerable to infections such as pneumonia.

Establishing an environment conducive to sleep requires adherence to a regular sleep routine, provision of comfortable sleeping space, and implementation of relaxation strategies before bed.

Additionally, limiting screen-based electronic device usage, such as that of smartphones and computers, at least one hour before bedtime can aid in sleep improvement.

Additionally, nutrition affects sleep hygiene. Specific food groups, including those abundant in tryptophan (found in nuts, seeds, and turkey), melatonin (found in cherries and grapes), and magnesium (found in leafy greens and nuts), have the potential to enhance the quality of sleep.

By promoting restful sleep, incorporating these foods into evening meals or snacks may help maintain a healthy immune system.

Management Of Stress To Prevent Pneumonia

There is evidence linking chronic stress to immune suppression, which increases susceptibility to infections. Stress management is an essential component of pneumonia prevention. Progressive muscle relaxation, mindfulness meditation, and deep breathing exercises are all effective methods that can be employed to alleviate stress and enhance general welfare.

Mental health can benefit from participation in pleasurable and calming activities, such as interests, time spent in nature, and socializing with loved ones. During periods of stress, sufficient social support is vital and can aid in the development of a robust immune system.

Furthermore, by including adaptogenic herbs in one's dietary regimen, such as holy basil and ashwagandha, the body may be better able to withstand stressors and maintain equilibrium. The anti-stress properties of these herbs have been revered in numerous cultures throughout history.

In summary, the Pneumonia Prevention Cookbook incorporates the aforementioned ideas into a comprehensive framework that promotes respiratory well-being. By prioritizing beverages that provide respiratory support, adhering to a healthy lifestyle that includes regular exercise and respiratory wellness, practicing good sleep hygiene, and managing stress effectively, individuals can actively mitigate the likelihood of contracting pneumonia and enhance their overall state of being. It is imperative to seek personalized advice from healthcare professionals or nutritionists, particularly in cases where pre-existing health conditions are present.

Conclusion

In summary, the Pneumonia Prevention Cookbook serves as an all-encompassing and indispensable manual for enhancing respiratory well-being via dietary decisions. This gastronomic manual adeptly combines the domains of preventative medicine and nutrition, providing an abundance of delectable recipes that are specifically formulated to strengthen the immune system and mitigate the risk of pneumonia.

This cookbook emphasizes the importance of ingredients that are abundant in nutrients and are recognized for their ability to enhance the immune system.

Emphasizing the integration of antioxidants, vitamins, and minerals, it offers a pragmatic strategy for enhancing resistance to respiratory infections. Through the integration of a wide range of fruits, vegetables, whole cereals, and lean proteins, the cookbook not only fortifies the body's immune system but also promotes holistic health.

Furthermore, the cookbook functions as more than a mere collection of recipes; it imparts knowledge to readers regarding the correlation between respiratory health and nutrition. Transparent elucidations regarding the advantages of particular constituents enable individuals to exercise agency in their dietary decisions, thereby cultivating a proactive stance toward the prevention of pneumonia.

Fundamentally, the Pneumonia Prevention Cookbook surpasses conventional gastronomic manuals by transforming into a comprehensive wellness companion.

By promoting a health-conscious and mindful approach to food, this initiative not only stimulates the senses but also enlightens individuals about the importance of incorporating respiratory health into their daily routines.

THE END

41

www.ingramcontent.com/pod-product-compliance
Lightning Source LLC
Chambersburg PA
CBHW050708250726
48662CB00002B/907